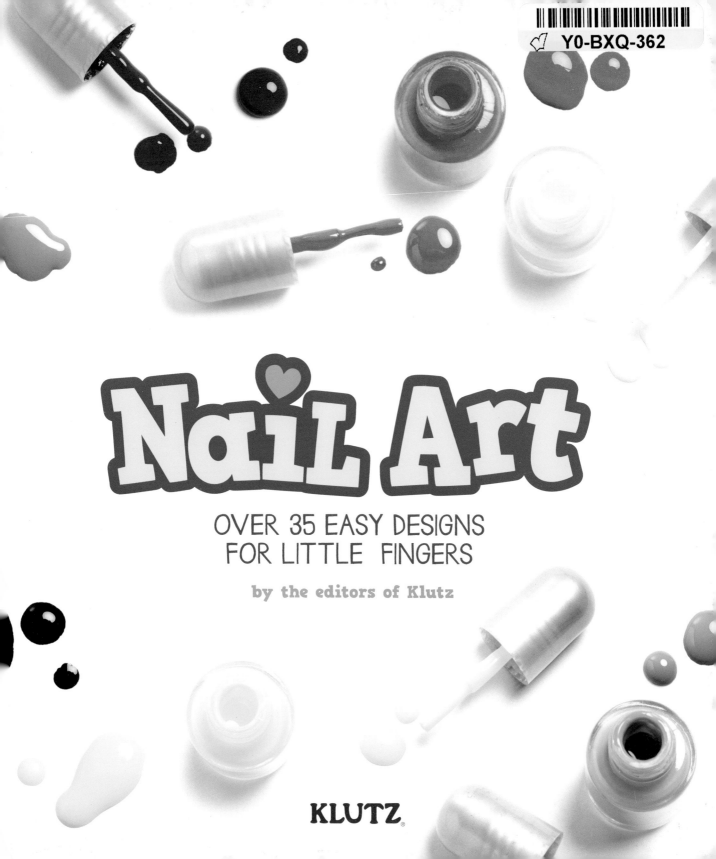

Nail Art

OVER 35 EASY DESIGNS
FOR LITTLE FINGERS

by the editors of Klutz

KLUTZ

CONTENTS

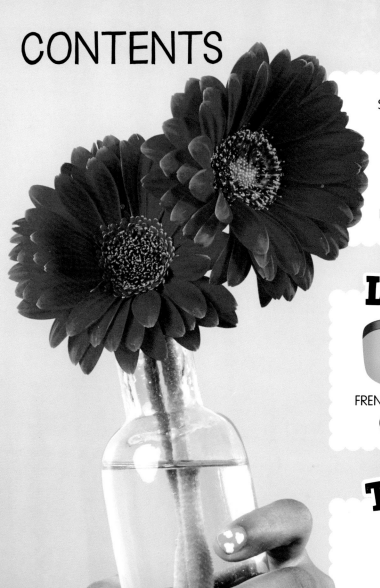

Creatures & Critters

COW
23

COW SPOTS
23

POOCH
24

PUPPY
25

PAW
25

KITTY
26

BEAR
28

BUNNY
29

CHICK
30

FISH
32

BUBBLES
33

STARFISH
34

HAPPY FACE
35

MONSTER
36

SPOTTED MONSTER
37

Garden

TULIP
39

DAISY
40

BLOSSOM
40

ROSEBUDS
41

RAINBOW
42

CLOUDS
43

LADYBUG
44

BEE
46

MUSHROOM
47

Party Time

BALLOON
49

FROSTING
50

BIRTHDAY GIRL
52

PARTY POOPER
53

BOW
54

TUX
55

WHAT YOU GET

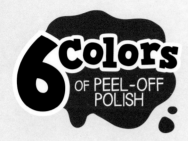
6 colors OF PEEL-OFF POLISH

This polish is non-toxic and specially designed to wash or peel off easily with warm water. That's so you can try a design, take it off, then try it again. If you want your design to last, ask an adult whether you can use regular nail polish (the kind you buy at the drugstore).

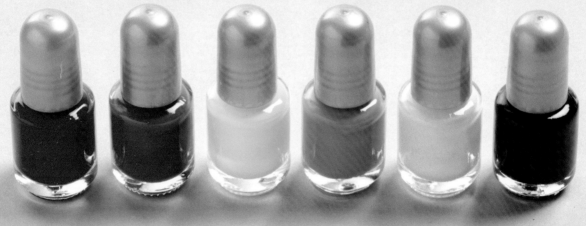

Detail Brush

What You Need

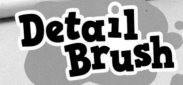

- A cup or bowl of water
- A paper towel
- A piece of paper

Before you begin your designs, paint one nail to make sure you don't have an allergic reaction. If you do develop a rash, remove the polish immediately with warm, soapy water. Go see your doctor if the problem continues. Don't paint over open wounds. And (obviously), don't eat the polish or give it to someone who might. If you spill the polish, clean up with water and soap.

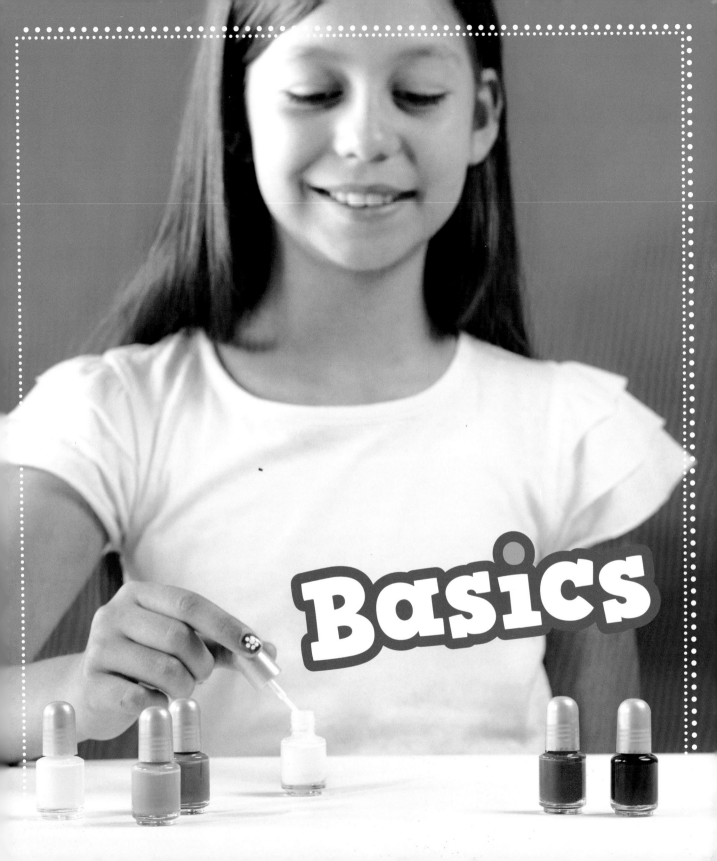

Basics

SETTING UP

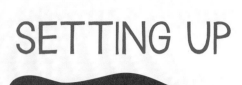

Having everything you need in one place will make painting your nails easier.

1 ADD A BOWL OF WATER

Fill a small bowl or cup halfway with water. You'll use this to clean the detail brush. Place a paper towel near the cup. Use this to dry the brush after you clean it.

2 PUT OUT THE POLISH

Arrange your polish so you can see all the colors. To prevent spills, put the cap on each bottle immediately after using it. Keep the polish a little away from you in case you forget to close the bottles.

3 STEADY THE BRUSH

The handle of your brush is round, which means it can roll away easily. Keep it on the paper towel or rest it against a closed polish bottle.

4 PUT OUT A PALETTE

Keep a paper palette near your brushes (see page 10).

GIVE YOURSELF A MANICURE

This quick manicure is a good way to prep your nails before you start a design. It's also okay to skip it if you want to start painting right away.

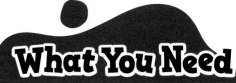

What You Need

- nail brush
- nail clippers
- file
- lotion

If you're wearing regular nail polish, you'll also need:

- cotton balls
- nail polish remover

1 CLEAN

Take off old polish. If you're wearing the polish that comes with this book, wash your nails with warm, soapy water and peel off the polish. Use the nail brush to clean under your nails.

TIP
Are you wearing regular nail polish? Use the cotton balls and polish remover to take it off.

2 TRIM

If your nails aren't the same length, trim them so they are even. Try for a nice rounded shape. If you need help, ask an adult.

3 FILE

Put the file just under the tip of your nail. Angle it away from your nail and make long, even strokes in one direction. Don't file back and forth.

Start on the left side and file toward the center. Then file from the right side toward the center.

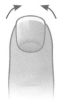

TIP
Filing can be tricky. Ask an adult if you need help.

4 LOTION

Rub some lotion on your hands. Wait for it to soak in (about ten minutes) before you begin your design.

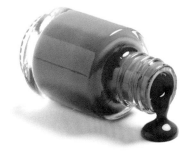

HOW TO PAINT YOUR NAILS

The key to a perfectly painted nail is using just the right amount of polish. Here's how...

1 Dip the brush into the bottle. Wipe all sides of the brush against the inside of the bottle lip to remove extra polish. The brush should be thinly coated, not globby.

 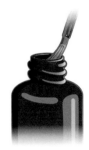

2 Paint a stripe in the middle of your nail. Begin at the bottom of your nail and move toward the tip.

3 Now paint the left side of your nail...

...and then the right side. Let the polish dry.

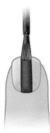

TIP
Keep your hand flat on the table while you work.

 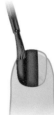 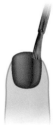

4 Some of the colors that come with this book (white and yellow) will need a second coat. After you add more polish, let it dry completely. Now you're ready to begin your design.

DRYING TIME
It usually takes about three to four minutes for the polish to dry. If you use a thicker coat, it will take longer.

To speed up drying, use a blow-dryer on the cool setting.

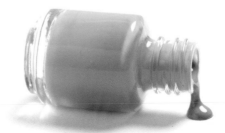

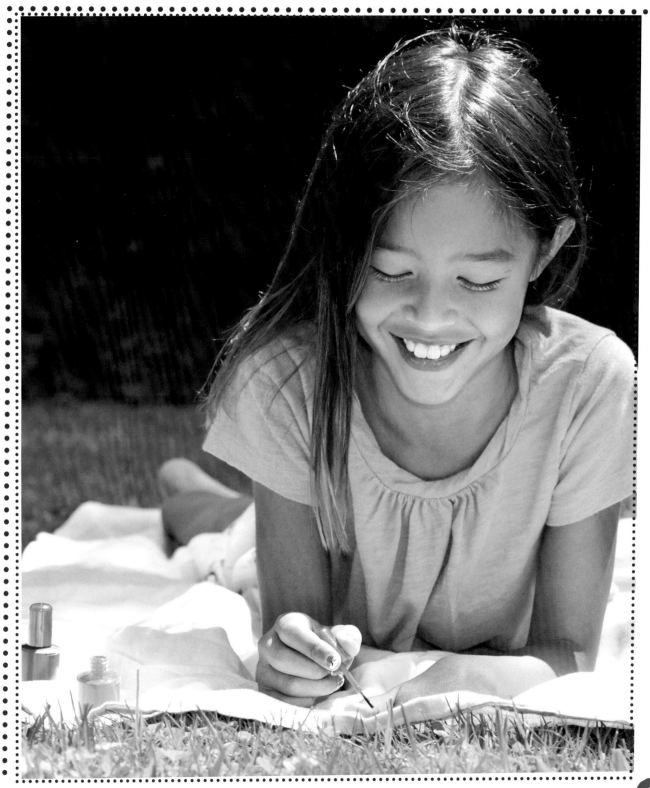

USING THE DETAIL BRUSH

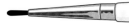

This is the detail brush.
You'll use it to make small details that are difficult to paint with the regular polish brush.

ADDING POLISH TO THE DETAIL BRUSH

The best way to add polish to the detail brush is to make a palette. Fold a piece of paper in half. Use the polish brush to put a drop of polish on the paper. Dip the detail brush in the drop whenever you need more polish.

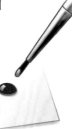

TIP
The polish will dry up after a bit, so make sure to add a new drop if it starts to get sticky.

PAINTING WITH THE DETAIL BRUSH

The key to using the detail brush is how much paint you use and how much pressure you apply.

TO MAKE BIG SHAPES
like these clouds…

…use a good amount of polish and more pressure.

TO MAKE SMALL DOTS, LINES, AND SHAPES
like the watermelon seeds and rind…

…use less polish and medium pressure.

TO MAKE TINY DOTS
like the black dot on the eye…

…use a tiny bit of polish and light pressure.

DOTTING TIPS

- *Gently touch the tip of the brush to your nail.*
- *Keep the brush straight up (don't tilt it to the side).*
- *Don't worry if your dots aren't perfect. Variation is pretty.*

Start using the detail brush when you see this:

…. NOW SWITCH TO …. THE DETAIL BRUSH

HELPFUL HINTS

COVER YOUR WORKSPACE

It's best to work on a flat surface, like a table or countertop. Lay down some butcher paper or newspaper before you begin.

AN EXTRA HAND

You'll probably need help painting one of your hands (the one you write with). Pair up with a friend or adult and take turns painting each other's nails.

YOUR NAILS

Your nails may look different from the ones you'll see in this book. That's okay – just play around with the designs to find the proportions that look best for you.

TIP
Keep your hand flat on your work surface while you design. This will make it easier to paint small details.

PRACTICE HELPS

It may be tricky to get some of these designs right the first, second, or even third time you do them. But with a little practice and some patience, your designs will look gorgeous in no time.

CLEANING THE BRUSH

For many of the designs, you'll use the detail brush with more than one color. Make sure to clean the brush in the water bowl and dry it before you dip it in a new color – and after you finish painting your nails.

TIP
Be gentle with the brush. Dip it into the water, don't press it against the bottom of the bowl.

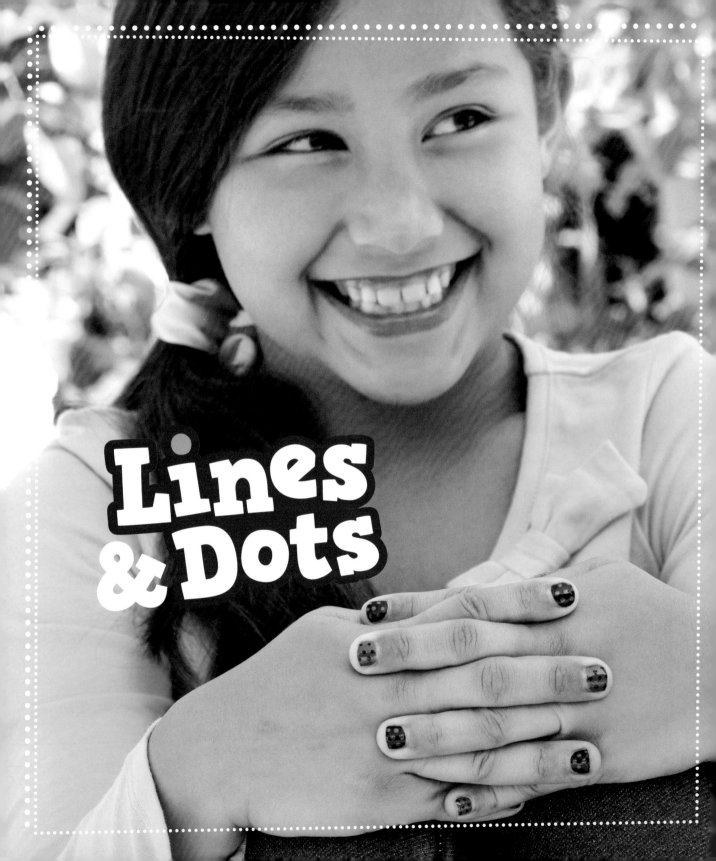

Lines & Dots

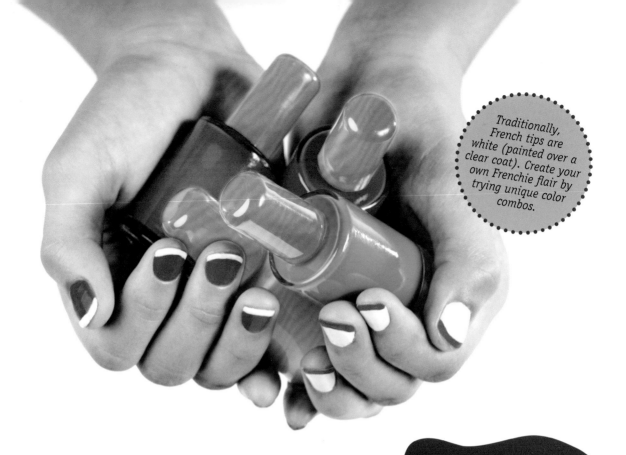

Traditionally, French tips are white (painted over a clear coat). Create your own Frenchie flair by trying unique color combos.

FRENCH TIPS

WHAT YOU NEED

Polish for the solid coat (any color you like)

Polish for the tips (also your choice)

1 Paint your nails with the solid color (you may need two coats). Wait for the polish to dry completely.

2 Now use the tip color to paint a curved line along the tip of your nail.

TIP
Painting French tips is tricky. Don't worry if it takes a while to get the hang of it. Just peel off the polish and try again.

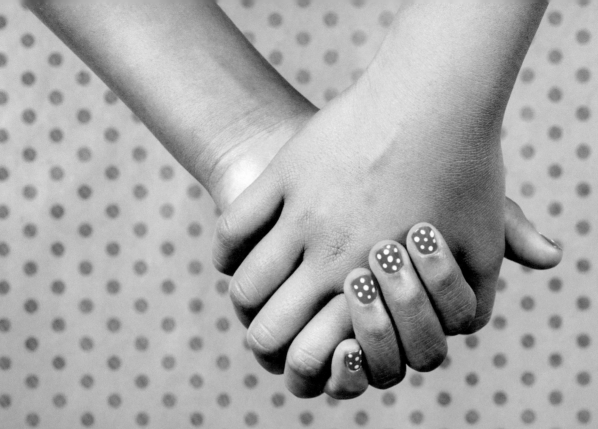

POLKA DOTS

WHAT YOU NEED

Polish for the solid coat (any color you like)

Polish for the dots (also your choice)

1

 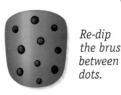

2

Re-dip the brush between dots.

Paint your nails with the solid color (you may need two coats). Wait for the polish to dry completely.

···· NOW SWITCH TO ····
THE DETAIL BRUSH

Make dots in the dot color, starting at the bottom of your nail and working your way up. See "Dotting Tips" on page 10.

TIP
Make sure you have a good amount of polish on your brush when dotting.

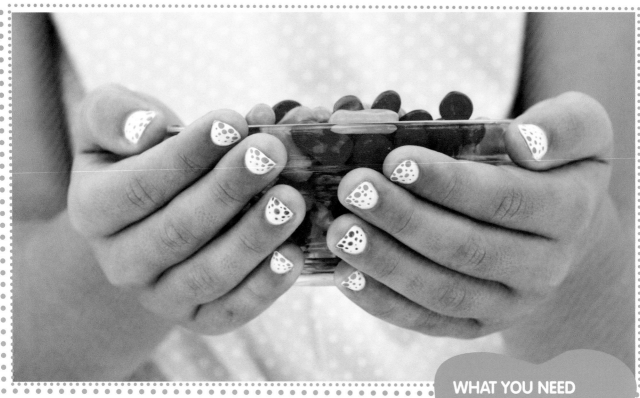

SPECKLES

WHAT YOU NEED

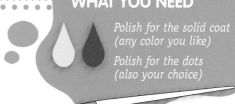

Polish for the solid coat
(any color you like)

Polish for the dots
(also your choice)

Paint your nails with
the solid color (you may
need two coats). Wait
for the polish to dry
completely.

.... NOW SWITCH TO ....
THE DETAIL BRUSH

*Re-dip
the brush
between
dots.*

Make lots of tiny dots
near the tip of your nail
in the second color. It's
okay if the dots overlap.

Add some more dots,
spacing them farther
apart as you move
down the nail.

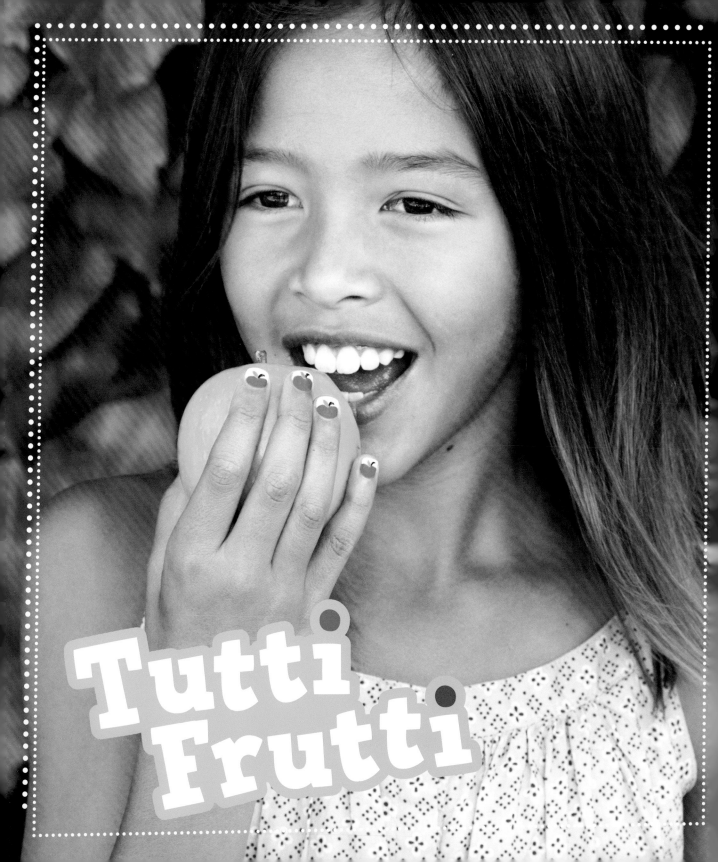

Tutti Frutti

WATERMELON

 1

Paint your nails pink. Wait for the polish to dry completely.

···· NOW SWITCH TO ···· THE DETAIL BRUSH

 2

Paint a curved teal line along the bottom edge of your nail.

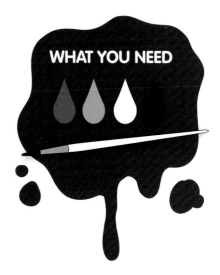

WHAT YOU NEED

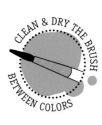

CLEAN & DRY THE BRUSH BETWEEN COLORS

 3

Paint a skinnier, curved white line right above the teal one.

TIP
If your nails are short, skip the white line and go straight to step 4.

 4

Make the outside seeds lean in toward the middle.

Paint three short black lines on the pink part of your nail. These are the seeds.

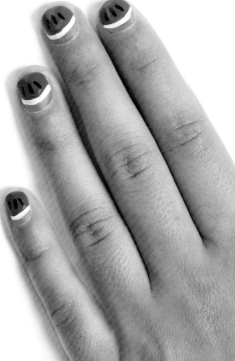

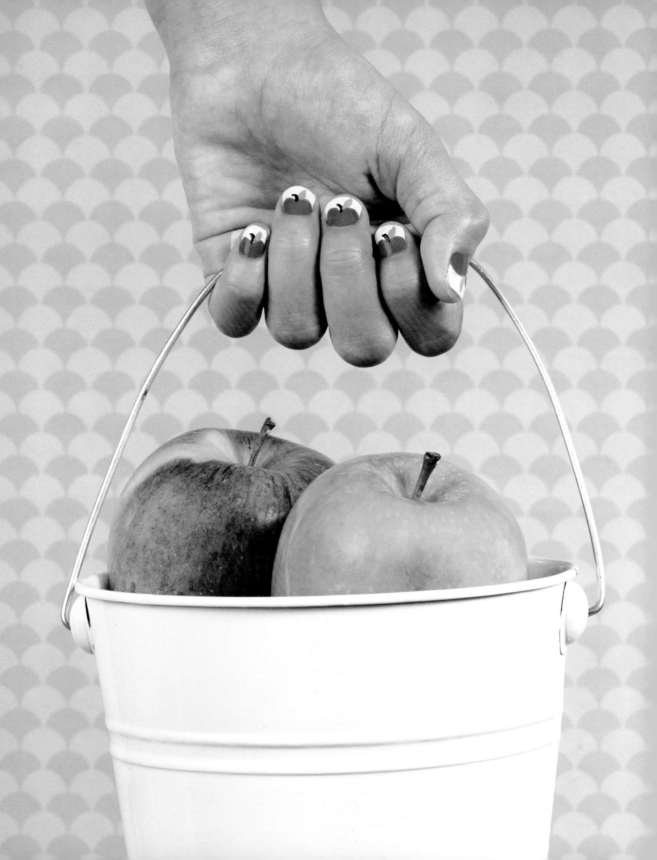

APPLE

WHAT YOU NEED

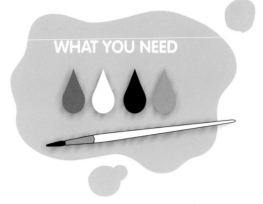

1

Paint your nails white. Let the polish dry, then add another coat. Wait for that coat to dry, too.

.... NOW SWITCH TO ....
THE DETAIL BRUSH

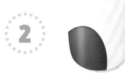

2

Paint a round coral shape on the left side of your nail, just like in the picture.

3

Make another round coral shape on the other side. Together, the shapes should look like the top of a heart. Let the polish dry.

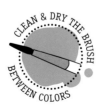

CLEAN & DRY THE BRUSH BETWEEN COLORS

4

Paint a small black line that curves to the left. This is the stem.

5

Add a teal leaf next to the stem.

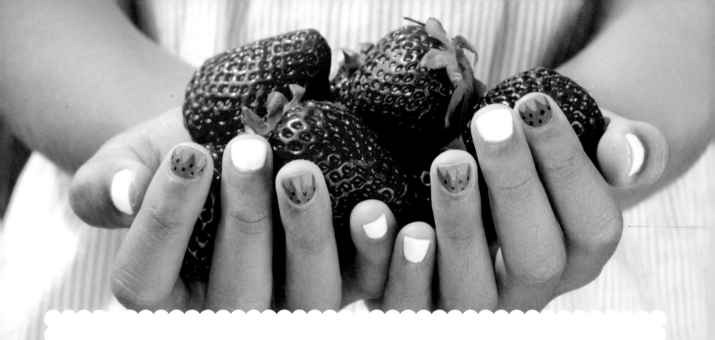

STRAWBERRY

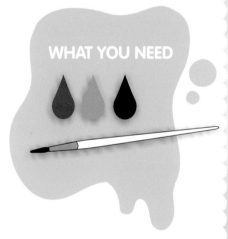

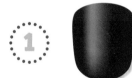 **1**

Paint your nails pink. Wait for the polish to dry completely.

···· NOW SWITCH TO ····
THE DETAIL BRUSH

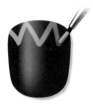 **2**

Make three V's on the tip of your nail: Coat the brush in teal and lay it down on your nail to make six short, angled lines.

 3

If you need to, fill in the V's with teal.

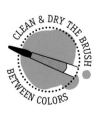

CLEAN & DRY THE BRUSH
BETWEEN COLORS

 4

Finish by adding seeds. Make small black dots on the pink part of your nail.

Re-dip the brush between dots.

GRAPEFRUIT

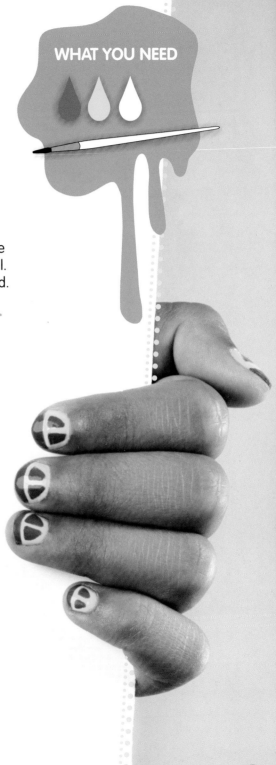

1 Paint your nails yellow. Let the polish dry, then add another coat. Wait for that coat to dry, too.

2 Paint a curved, coral line along the tip of your nail. This is the grapefruit rind.

.... NOW SWITCH TO ....
THE DETAIL BRUSH

3 Make a coral triangle on the left side of your nail.

Try to make the top of the shape curved, just like the coral tip.

4 Paint another coral triangle on the right side of your nail.

TIP
Change the size of the triangles to fit the shape of your nails.

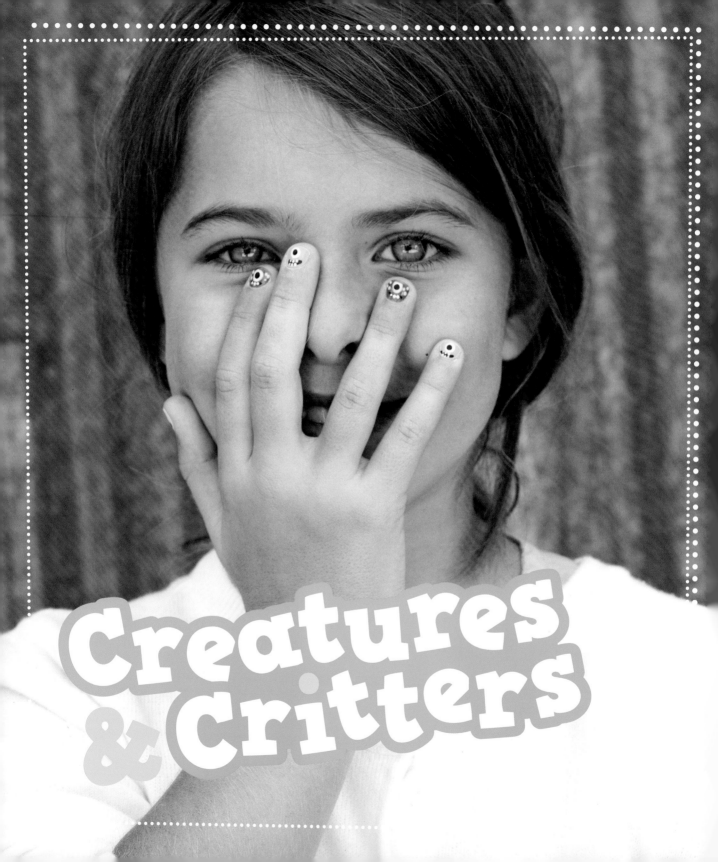

Creatures
& Critters

COW

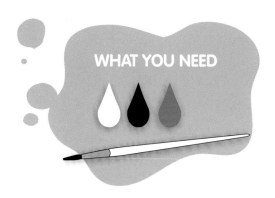
 1

Paint your nails white. Let the polish dry, then add another coat. Wait for that coat to dry, too.

.... NOW SWITCH TO ....
THE DETAIL BRUSH

 2

Paint a coral oval at the bottom of your nail. Wait for the polish to dry.

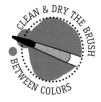

CLEAN & DRY THE BRUSH
BETWEEN COLORS

 3

The nostrils should angle in a little.

Make two short black lines for nostrils and two black dots for eyes.

 4

Paint four black blobs around the edge of your nail. Spots!

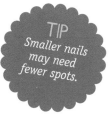

TIP
Smaller nails may need fewer spots.

COW SPOTS

Try painting the cow on one nail, then paint these spectacular spots on the rest.

Cover your whole nail with spots.

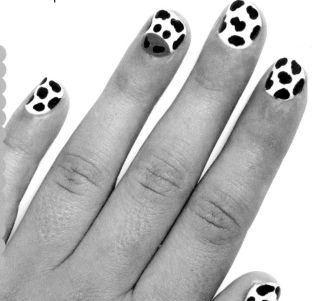

23

POOCH

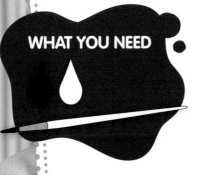

WHAT YOU NEED

Paint your nails black. Wait for the polish to dry completely.

.... NOW SWITCH TO ....
THE DETAIL BRUSH

Paint a white triangle at the bottom of your nail.

Now paint a white stripe from the top of the triangle to the tip of your nail. Wait for all the white to dry.

Follow the steps below to make the eyes.

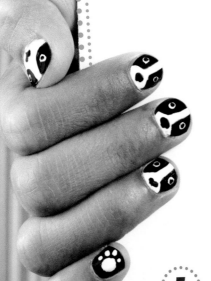

To make the nose, paint a small black heart near the bottom of your nail.

HOW TO MAKE EYES

Make two small white dots. Let them dry. Clean the detail brush.

Add a tiny black dot on top of each white dot.

PUPPY

Turn your pooch into a pup with just a few small changes.

Paint your nail with two coats of teal. After it dries, add a taller white triangle.

Now, make a big white spot on the top left side of your nail. Let all the white dry.

Make two black dots for eyes. Next, add the heart nose.

PAW

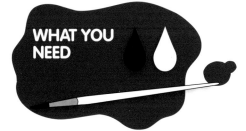

WHAT YOU NEED

Paint your nails black. Wait for the polish to dry completely.

.... NOW SWITCH TO ....
THE DETAIL BRUSH

Paint a white circle near the bottom corner of your nail. Then add four small ovals around the top half of the circle.

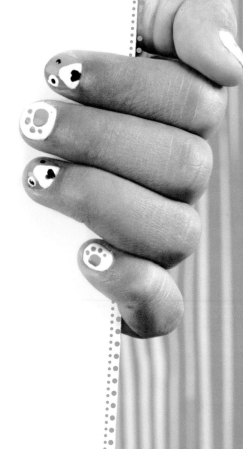

KITTY

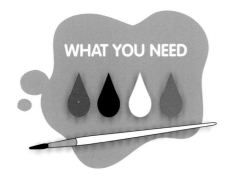

WHAT YOU NEED

Paint your nails pink. Wait for the polish to dry completely.

.... NOW SWITCH TO ....
THE DETAIL BRUSH

Leave some space between the circle and the tip of your nail.

Paint an off-center black circle near the bottom of your nail. Wait for the polish to dry.

Add two black triangles for ears.

TIP
Use only a little polish when painting details like the ears and tail.

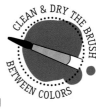

CLEAN & DRY THE BRUSH BETWEEN COLORS

Paint a thin black line along the left side of your nail. Make the tail curl in at the end.

Make two eyes (see "How to Make Eyes" on page 24).

Make a small coral dot for the nose.

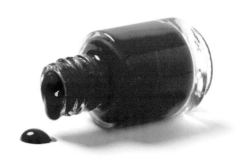

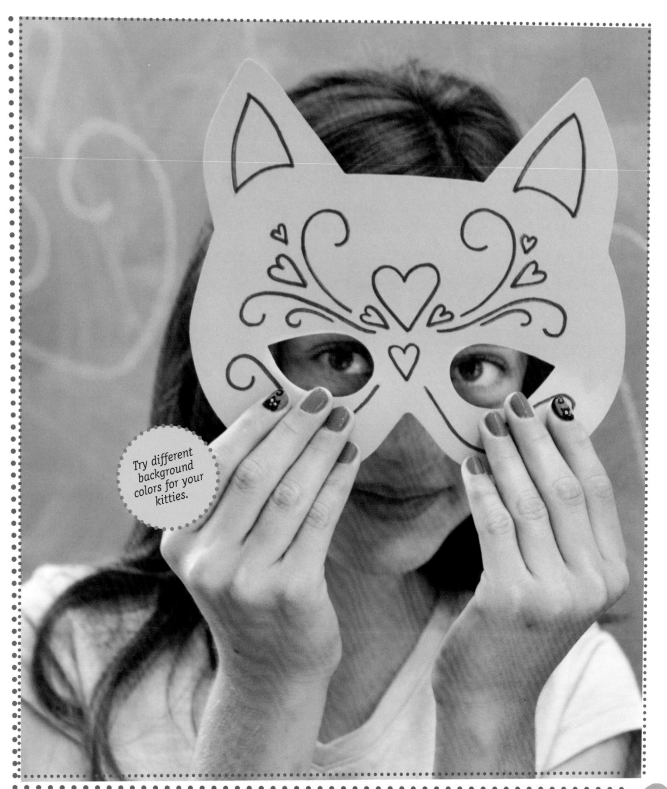

Try different background colors for your kitties.

BEAR

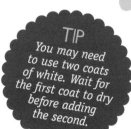

1

Paint your nails black. Wait for the polish to dry completely.

.... NOW SWITCH TO ....
THE DETAIL BRUSH

2

To make the bear's head, paint a big white circle at the bottom of your nail.

TIP
You may need to use two coats of white. Wait for the first coat to dry before adding the second.

3

Add two small white circles for ears. Wait for all the white to dry.

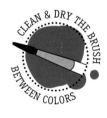

CLEAN & DRY THE BRUSH
BETWEEN COLORS

4

Make the eyes pretty far apart.

Now make two short black lines for eyes and a small black dot for the nose. Use only a tiny bit of polish.

Try different background colors for your bears.

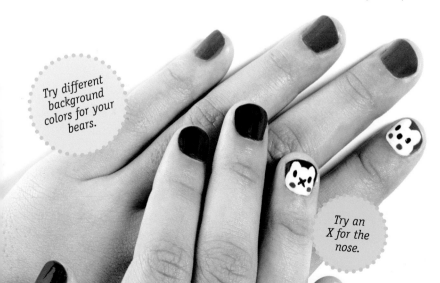

Try an X for the nose.

5

To make cheeks, use the detail brush to paint two big pink dots below the eyes.

BUNNY

Try these easy tweaks to transform the bear into a bunny.

 1
Make the bunny head a little shorter than the bear head.

 2
Make the ears longer and closer together.

 3
Give the bunny the same face as the bear.

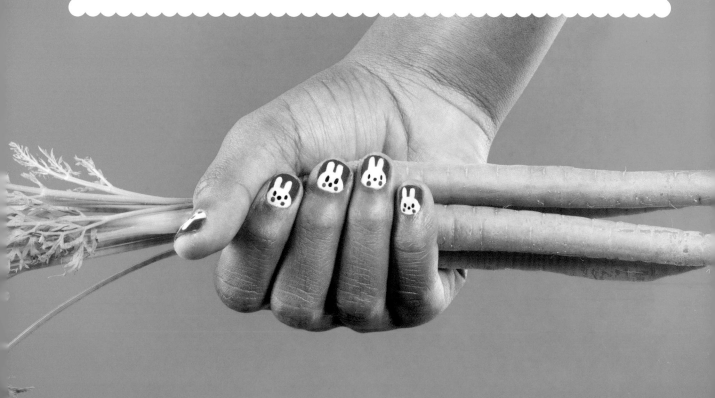

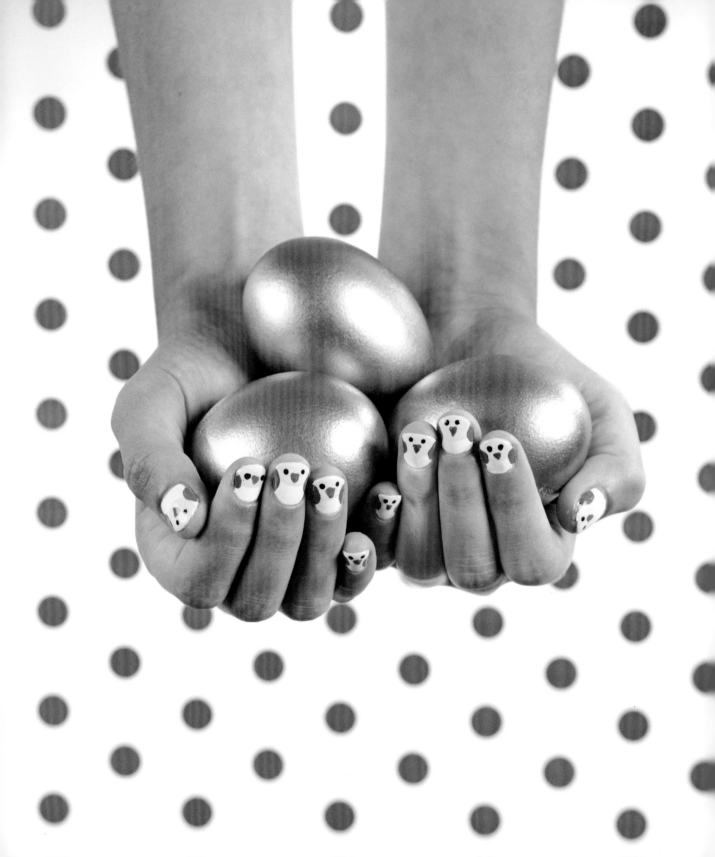

CHICK

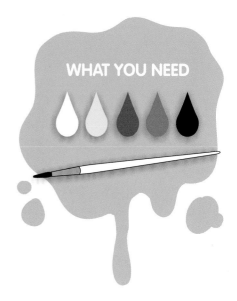

1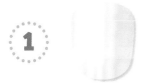

Paint your nails white. Let the polish dry, then add another coat. Wait for that coat to dry, too.

.... NOW SWITCH TO ....
THE DETAIL BRUSH

2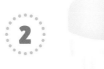

Paint the top half of your nail yellow. This is the chick's head. Wait for the polish to dry.

3

Try to make the wings about the same size.

Paint two pink half ovals, one on each side of your nail. Wings!

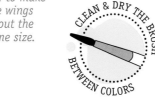

CLEAN & DRY THE BRUSH
BETWEEN COLORS

4

Make a tiny coral triangle for the beak.

5

Add two black dots for the eyes.

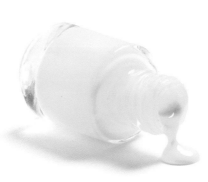

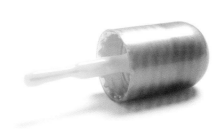

FISH

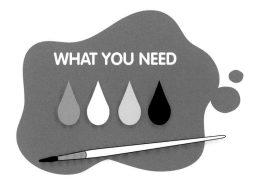

WHAT YOU NEED

 1

Paint your nails teal. Wait for the polish to dry completely.

.... NOW SWITCH TO ....
THE DETAIL BRUSH

 2

Paint a yellow oval near the middle of your nail.

 3

CLEAN & DRY THE BRUSH BETWEEN COLORS

Make two short yellow lines for the fish tail. Wait for the polish to dry.

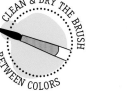

4

Make a black dot for the eye.

 5

Re-dip the brush between dots.

Use the detail brush to make white dots around the fish. Bubbles!

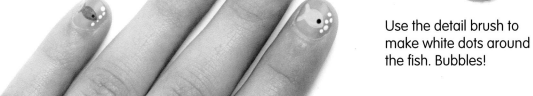

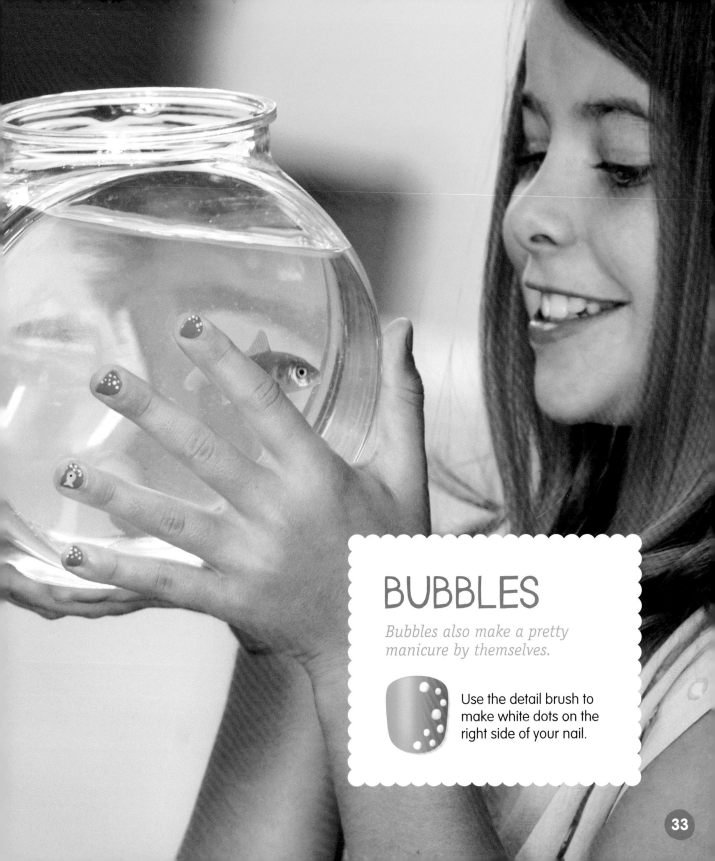

BUBBLES

Bubbles also make a pretty manicure by themselves.

Use the detail brush to make white dots on the right side of your nail.

STARFISH

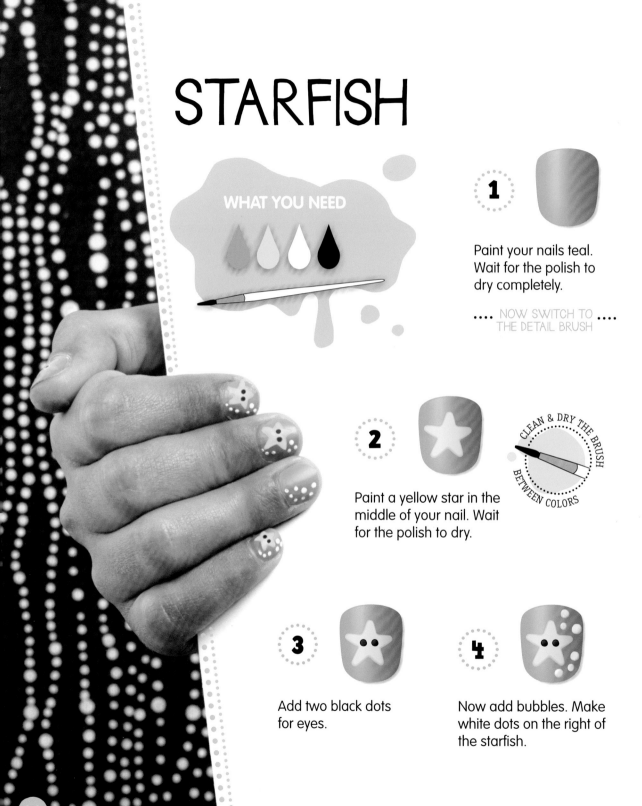

WHAT YOU NEED

1

Paint your nails teal.
Wait for the polish to
dry completely.

.... NOW SWITCH TO ....
THE DETAIL BRUSH

2

Paint a yellow star in the
middle of your nail. Wait
for the polish to dry.

CLEAN & DRY THE BRUSH
BETWEEN COLORS

3

Add two black dots
for eyes.

4

Now add bubbles. Make
white dots on the right of
the starfish.

HAPPY FACE

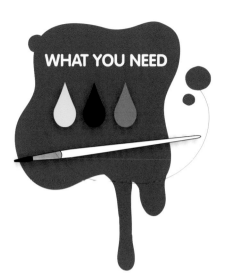

 1

Paint your nails yellow. Let the polish dry, then add another coat. Wait for that coat to dry, too.

.... NOW SWITCH TO ....
THE DETAIL BRUSH

 2

Make two black dots near the top of your nail.

Space the dots about this far apart.

 3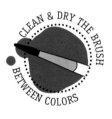

CLEAN & DRY THE BRUSH
BETWEEN COLORS

Make a curved line for a smile.

 4

If you want, paint two coral dots, one on either side of the smile. Rosy cheeks!

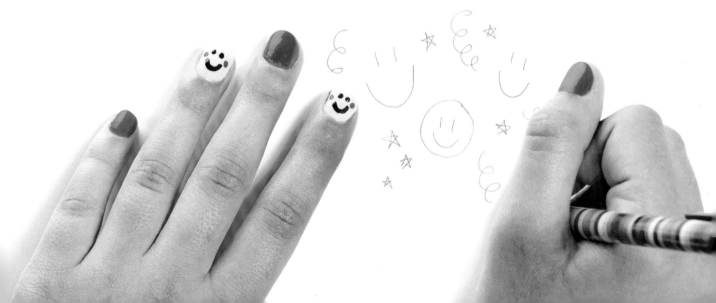

MONSTER

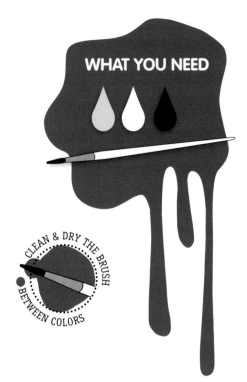

CLEAN & DRY THE BRUSH BETWEEN COLORS

1 Paint your nails yellow. Let the polish dry, then add another coat. Wait for that coat to dry, too.

.... NOW SWITCH TO THE DETAIL BRUSH

2 Make a black blob for the monster's mouth. Let it dry.

3 Paint a big white circle for the monster's eye.

4 Make tiny dots for teeth: three at the top of the mouth, four at the bottom. Wait for all the white to dry.

For an extra-goofy monster, vary the size of the teeth.

5 Make a big black dot in the middle of the eye.

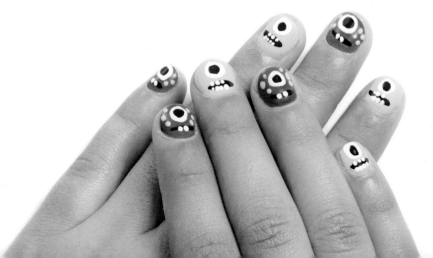

SPOTTED MONSTER

Monster makeover! Get a different beastly look by following these steps.

Give the monster the same eye. For the mouth, make a stripe instead of a blob.

Add only two teeth.

Re-dip the brush between dots.

Make yellow spots on the monster's face.

Try different background colors for your monsters.

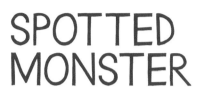
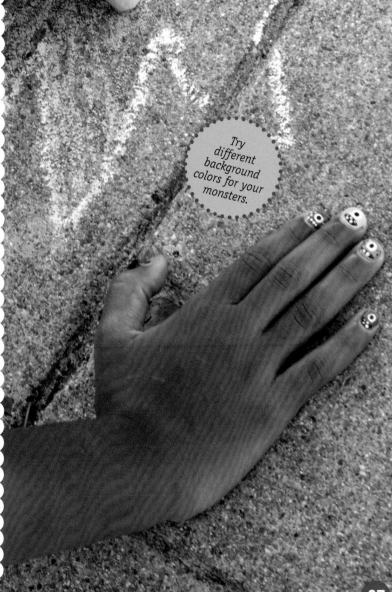

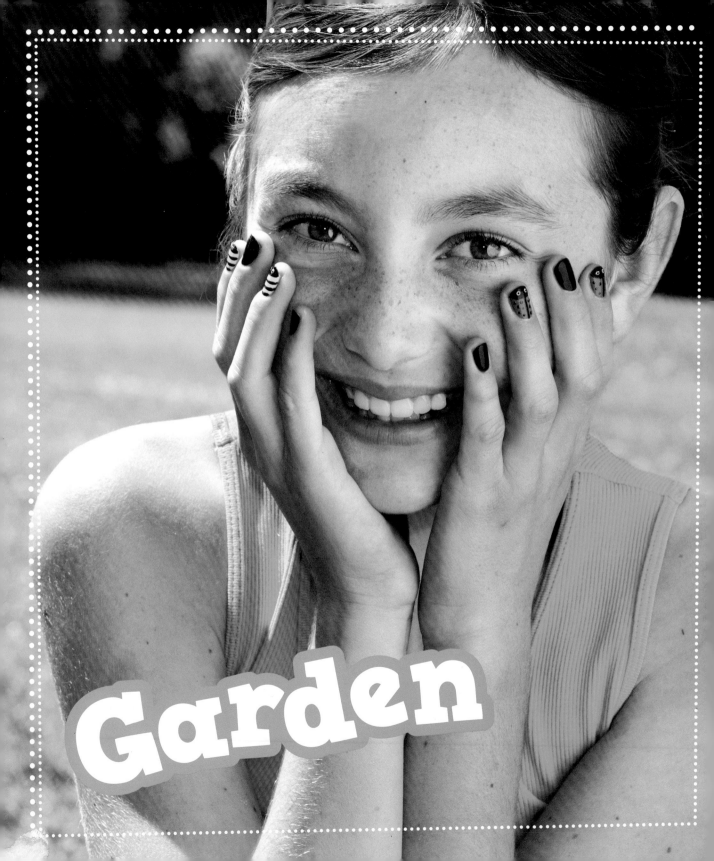

Garden

TULIP

1

Paint your nails pink. Wait for the polish to dry completely.

···· NOW SWITCH TO ····
THE DETAIL BRUSH

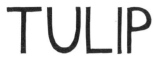

WHAT YOU NEED

2

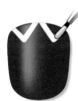

The two V's should meet in the middle of your nail.

Now make two V's on the tip of your nail: Coat the brush in white and lay it down on your nail to make four short, angled lines.

3

TIP
You may need to add a couple coats of white so the triangles look nice and crisp.

Fill in the V's with white. Beautiful!

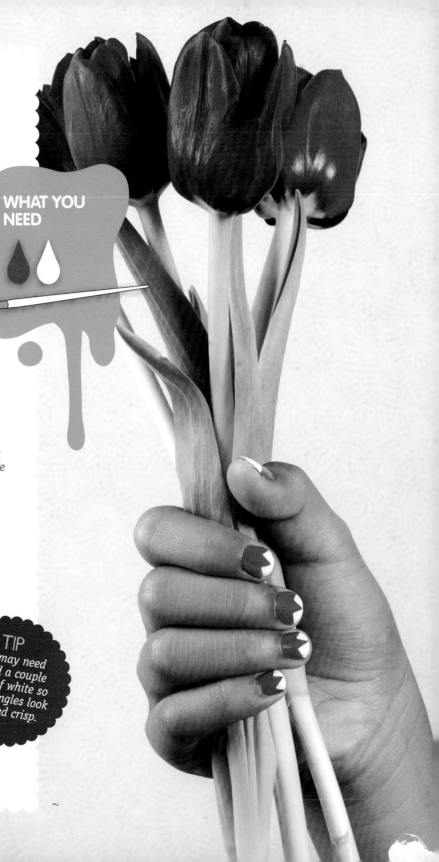

DAISY

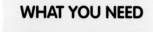

WHAT YOU NEED

1 Paint your nails teal. Wait for the polish to dry completely.

.... NOW SWITCH TO ....
THE DETAIL BRUSH

2 Use the detail brush to make a big yellow dot near the middle of your nail.

CLEAN & DRY THE BRUSH
BETWEEN COLORS

3 *It's okay if the dots overlap a little.*

Make five big white dots around the yellow one. Re-dip the brush after each dot.

BLOSSOM

It's easy to transform the daisy into a blossom.

1 Make all yellow dots. Space them farther from the center dot.

2 Connect the outside dots to the middle dot with little lines.

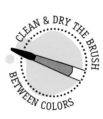

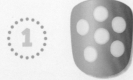

Try a different background color for your flowers.

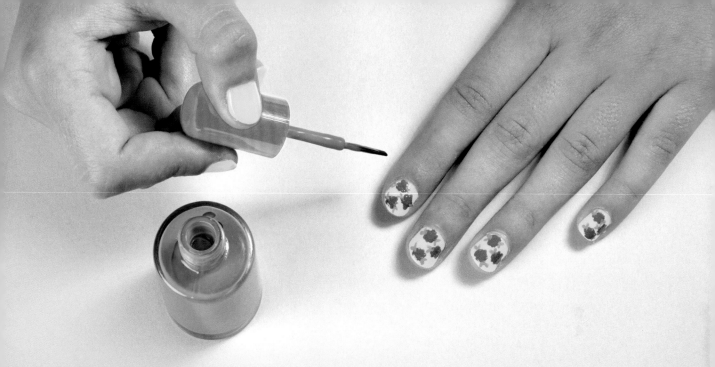

ROSEBUDS

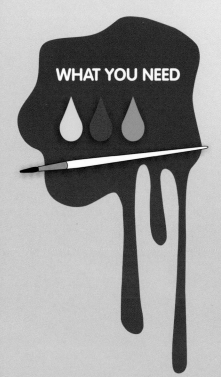

WHAT YOU NEED

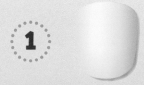

1

Paint your nails yellow.
Let the polish dry, then add
another coat. Wait for that
coat to dry, too.

···· NOW SWITCH TO ····
THE DETAIL BRUSH

2

Make three small pink
blobs on your nail.

CLEAN & DRY THE BRUSH
BETWEEN COLORS

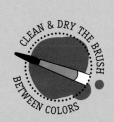

3

*Leave some
space between
the rosebuds.*

Now, make little teal V's on
the sides of the rosebuds.
These are the leaves.

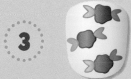

WHAT YOU NEED

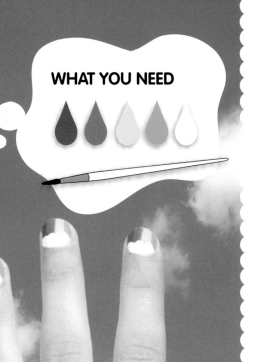

RAINBOW

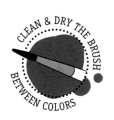
CLEAN & DRY THE BRUSH BETWEEN COLORS

1 Use the detail brush to paint a pink stripe down the side of your nail.

2 Paint three more stripes: coral, then yellow, and last teal. Let the polish dry completely.

3

The cloud should have three humps.

Make a big white blob for the cloud. You may need to use two coats of white.

CLOUDS

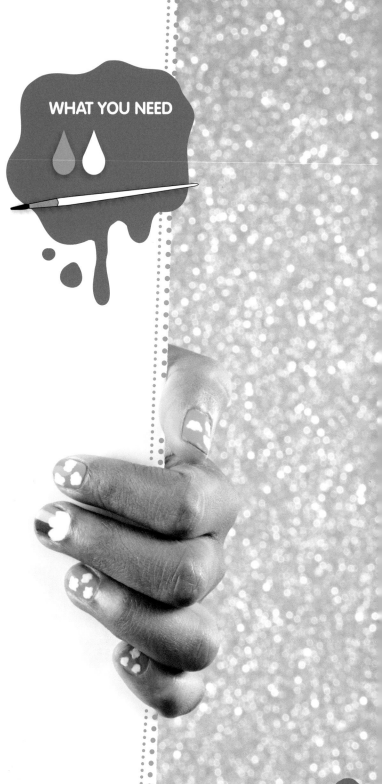

1

Paint your nails teal.
Wait for the polish to
dry completely.

···· NOW SWITCH TO ····
THE DETAIL BRUSH

2

Make a small white blob
on your nail.

3

*You may need
to use two coats
of white.*

Add two more white blobs.

43

LADYBUG

WHAT YOU NEED
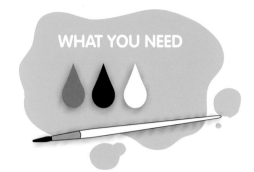

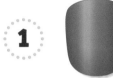

1 Paint your nails coral. Wait for the polish to dry completely.

...... NOW SWITCH TO ......
THE DETAIL BRUSH

2 Paint a black oval on the tip of your nail.

3 Paint a black stripe down the middle of your nail.

4 Make small black dots on the coral part of your nail.

Re-dip the brush between dots.

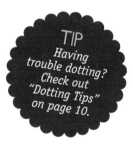

TIP
Having trouble dotting? Check out "Dotting Tips" on page 10.

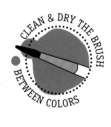

CLEAN & DRY THE BRUSH BETWEEN COLORS

5 Make two eyes (see "How to Make Eyes" on page 24).

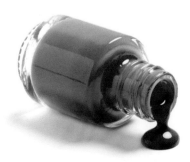

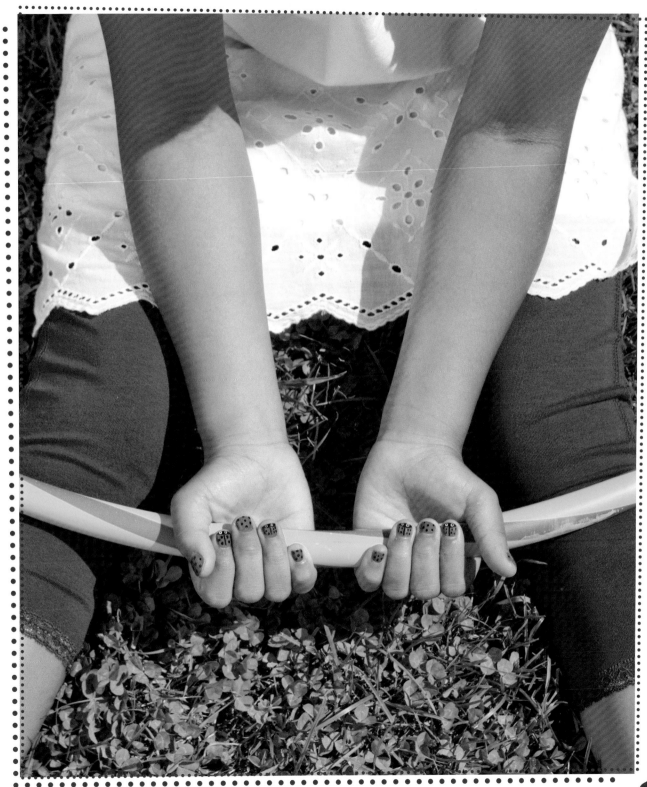

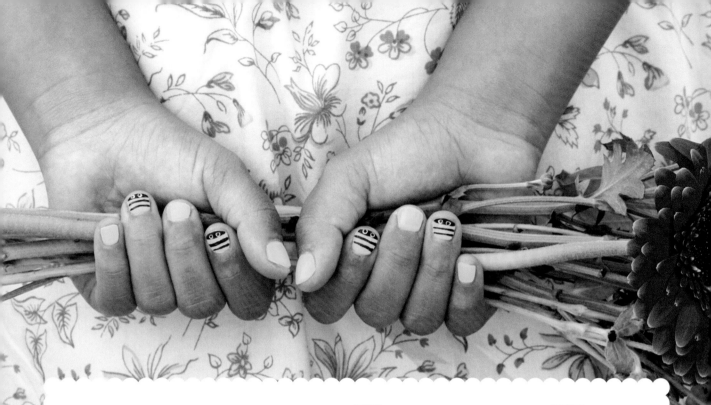

BEE

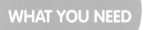
WHAT YOU NEED

①

Paint your nails yellow. Let the polish dry, then add another coat. Wait for that coat to dry, too.

.... NOW SWITCH TO ....
THE DETAIL BRUSH

②

Paint a black oval on the tip of your nail.

③

Paint two curved black lines across your nail. Wait for all the black to dry.

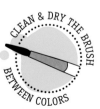
CLEAN & DRY THE BRUSH BETWEEN COLORS

④

Make two eyes (see "How to Make Eyes" on page 24).

MUSHROOM

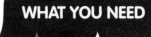
WHAT YOU NEED

Paint your nails coral.
Wait for the polish to
dry completely.

.... NOW SWITCH TO ....
THE DETAIL BRUSH

Paint a white oval
at the bottom of
your nail.

TIP
You may need
to use two coats
of white. Wait for
the first coat to dry
before adding
the second.

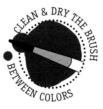
CLEAN & DRY THE BRUSH
BETWEEN COLORS

Make white dots above
the oval. Wait for all the
white to dry.

Now make two short black
lines for eyes. Use only
a tiny bit of polish.

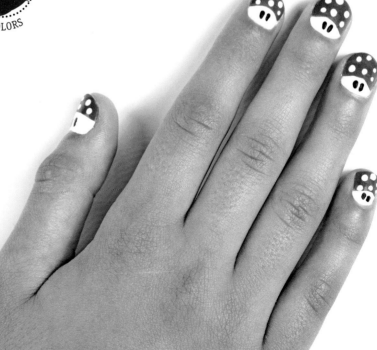

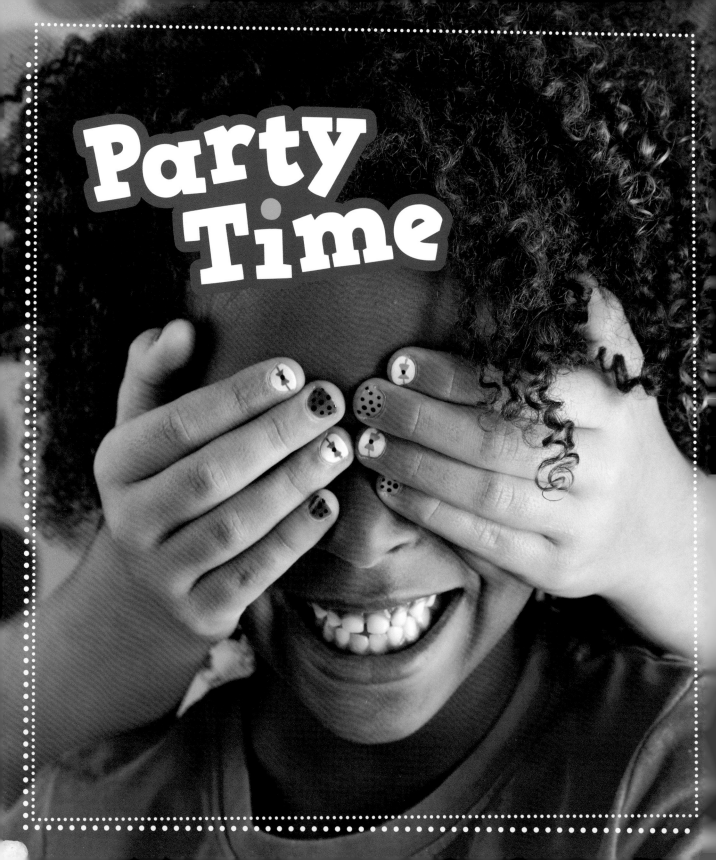

Party Time

BALLOON

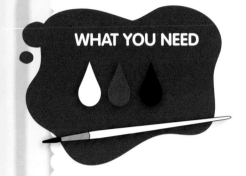

WHAT YOU NEED

1

Paint your nails white. Let the polish dry, then add another coat. Wait for that coat to dry, too.

.... NOW SWITCH TO ....
THE DETAIL BRUSH

2

Paint a round pink shape at the top of your nail. This is the balloon.

3

Make a small pink triangle at the bottom of the balloon.

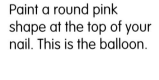
CLEAN & DRY THE BRUSH BETWEEN COLORS

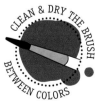

4

For the balloon string, make a curvy black line.

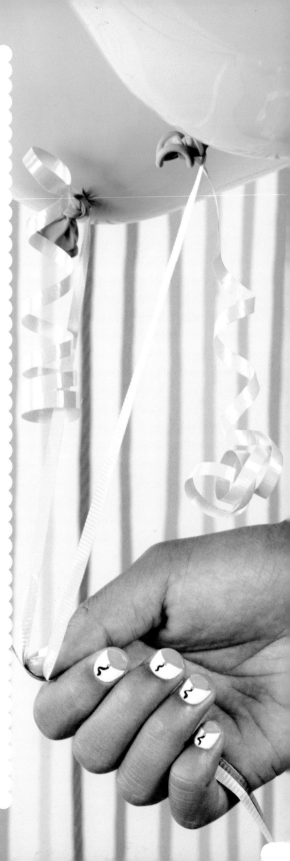

FROSTING

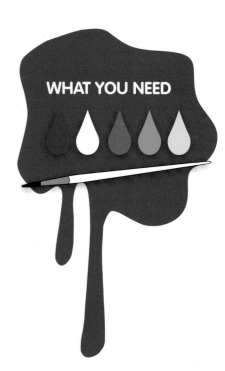

 1

Paint your nails pink. Wait for the polish to dry completely.

.... NOW SWITCH TO ....
THE DETAIL BRUSH

 2

You may need two coats of white.

Paint a drippy white shape on the top half of your nail. This is the frosting. Wait for the polish to dry.

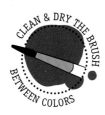
CLEAN & DRY THE BRUSH
BETWEEN COLORS

 3

Re-dip the brush between dots.

Use the detail brush to make a few small coral dots on the frosting. Sprinkles!

 4

Add some yellow and teal sprinkles, too.

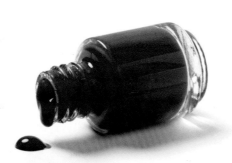

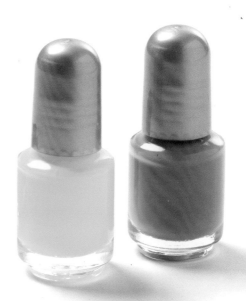

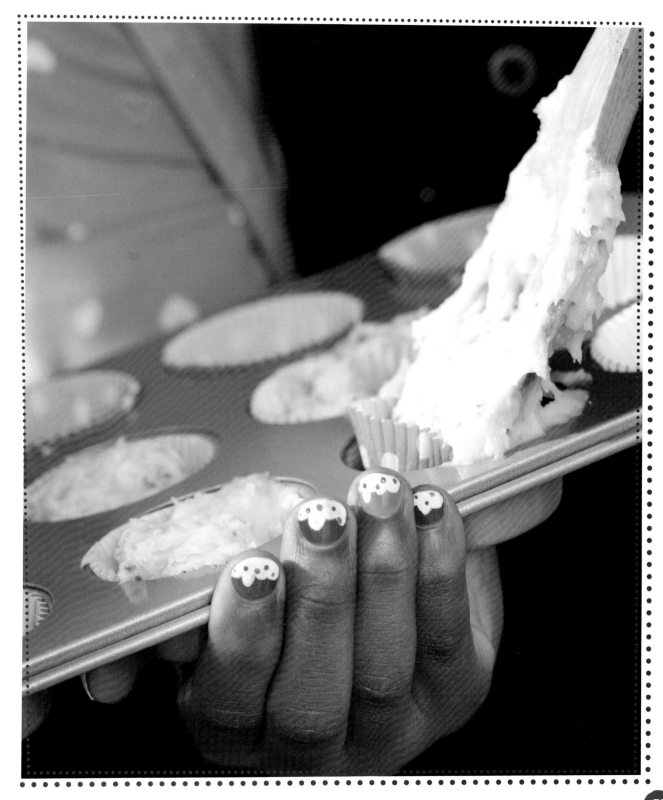

BIRTHDAY GIRL

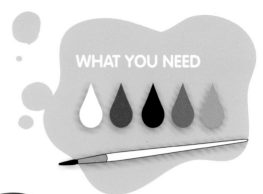

Paint your nails with two coats of white. Wait for the polish to dry completely.

.... NOW SWITCH TO ....
THE DETAIL BRUSH

Paint pink hair around the edge of your nail. Wait for the polish to dry.

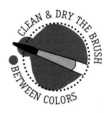

CLEAN & DRY THE BRUSH
BETWEEN COLORS

To get a thin line, use only a tiny bit of polish.

Make two small black dots for eyes. Then add a curved line for the smile.

Add two coral dots for cheeks.

If you want, make two curved blue lines for barrettes.

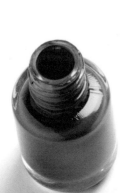
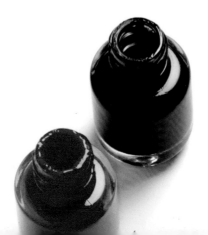
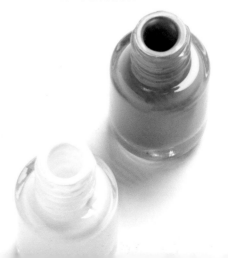

PARTY POOPER

Turn that birthday smile upside down to make this adorably grumpy girl.

Paint your nail with two coats of white. Let it dry, then add black hair.

Make two curved black lines for eyes. Use only a tiny bit of paint.

Paint a curved pink line for the frown.

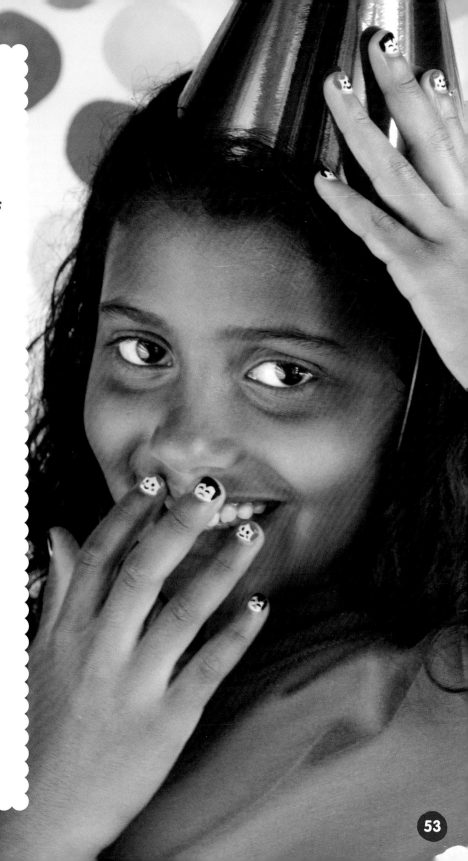

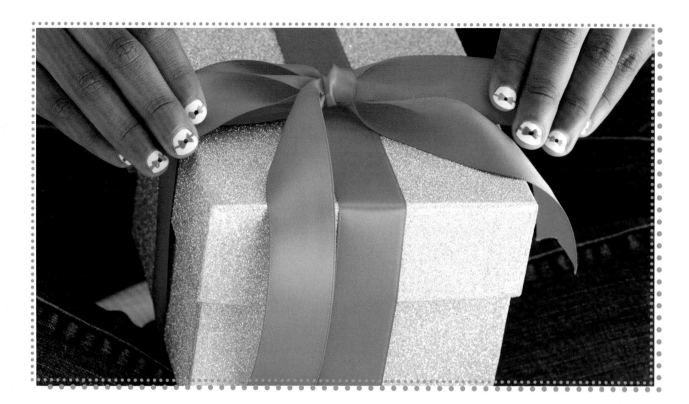

BOW

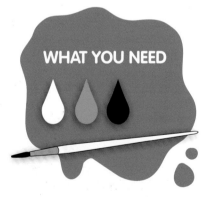

WHAT YOU NEED

1

Paint your nails white. Let the polish dry, then add another coat. Wait for that coat to dry, too.

···· NOW SWITCH TO ····
THE DETAIL BRUSH

2

In the middle of your nail, make two tiny teal triangles that touch.

3

Now paint two short teal lines on either side of the bow. Wait for the teal to dry.

CLEAN & DRY THE BRUSH
BETWEEN COLORS

4

Add a small black dot in the middle of the bow.

TUX

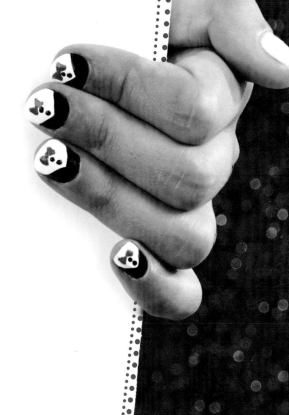

Paint your nails black. Wait for the polish to dry completely.

.... NOW SWITCH TO ....
THE DETAIL BRUSH

Paint a white upside-down triangle at the top of your nail. Wait for the polish to dry.

The bow tie should be near the tip of your nail.

Add a pink bow tie: Make two tiny triangles that touch.

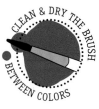

CLEAN & DRY THE BRUSH
BETWEEN COLORS

Make two small black dots below the bow tie. These are the shirt buttons.

CREDITS

EDITOR
Eva Steele-Saccio

ART DIRECTOR
Dirty Bandits

PRODUCT DIRECTOR
April Chorba

INSTRUCTIONAL ILLUSTRATOR
Jim Kopp

PHOTOGRAPHERS
Rory Earnshaw, John Lee

PACKAGE DESIGNER
David Avidor

PRODUCTION COORDINATOR
Kelly Beltramo

MANICURISTS
Shakira Holmes, Lily Huang,
Tinee Mahoney

SPECIAL THANKS
Rebekah Piatte

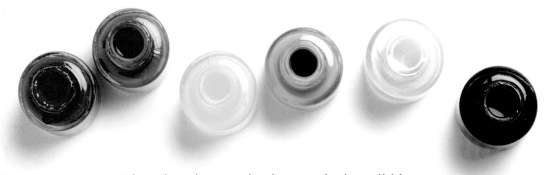

Here are more Klutz books we think your kids will like.

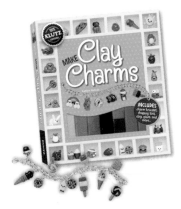

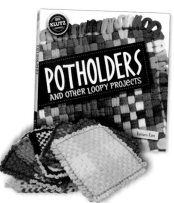

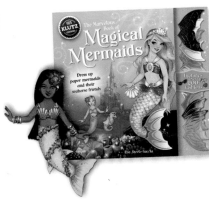

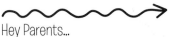